KETOGENIC DIET

50 Easy Recipes for Healthy Eating, Healthy Living & Weight Loss

Modern Kitchen

TABLE OF CONTENTS

INTRODUCTION

This book contains helpful facts about the ketogenic diet. It will help you understand the basics and benefits of the diet. It has simple steps and tips to get you through the diet. It also contains tasty and easy-to-do keto recipes you'll enjoy.

History of the Ketogenic Diet

The use of fasting to treat certain diseases, including epilepsy, can be traced to the physicians of ancient times. But because prolonged fasting often results in muscle loss and nutrient deficiencies, doctors eventually began to study modified diets. During the early 1920s, Dr. Russel Wilder developed the ketogenic diet and used it to treat epileptics. It remained a popular treatment for epilepsy, especially in children, through the next decade. But when improved anticonvulsant medications were developed around 1940, the use of ketogenic diets declined.

In 1994, the ketogenic diet regained its popularity thanks to Charlie Abrahams, a boy who suffered from epilepsy despite using anticonvulsant medications and other medical treatments. His seizures were controlled only through the implementation of the ketogenic diet. This inspired his father, Hollywood producer Jim Abrahams, to set up the Charlie Foundation, which promotes and funds research about the diet. Since then, further studies have been made, and less restrictive models have become available for people seeking general health improvement and also for those desiring weight loss.

Mechanism of the Ketogenic Diet

A typical modern diet is high in carbohydrates. That causes the body to use glucose as its primary source of energy. Fats, macronutrients that normally serve as an energy source, are therefore not used and are instead stored. On the other hand, the ketogenic diet's high-fat, moderate-protein, low-carbohydrate program causes the body to turn to fats as its energy source. Because of the lack of carbs, the liver will convert stored fats into ketone bodies and release them into the blood. These will then be used as fuel instead of the glucose from carbs. This metabolic state is called ketosis. When your body is in ketosis, fats are easily consumed rather than stored. That's why it is also called the "fat-burning mode" of the body. Ketosis is a normal result of staying on a low-carb diet (or of prolonged fasting or starvation).

Different enzymes are used for breaking down carbs and fats. Therefore, a body that is used to a high-carb diet will have to adjust before entering into ketosis. This may take three to four days. Before building up a new supply of enzymes, the body will first use up all the glucose that is left, resulting in weakness and lethargy. But once the body has adapted to ketosis, it will be able to maximize the use of fats. Some advocates of the keto diet even testify that they experience longer lasting energy throughout the day.

Is Ketosis dangerous?

Ketosis is often feared due to the confusion between it and ketoacidosis. If ketosis is the body's normal response to a low-carb diet, ketoacidosis is an abnormal condition where excessive ketone bodies in the bloodstream have overwhelmed the body's homeostasis – the compensatory mechanisms of the body – resulting in acidic blood pH. Ketosis is rumored to lead to ketoacidosis because ketone bodies are acidic. However, ketoacidosis actually results from a shortage of insulin, and is not due to a prolonged state of ketosis. So the only people at risk for ketoacidosis are those with type 1 diabetes or pancreatic disorders.

Food list

A keto diet is basically increasing your dietary fat intake, choosing low-carb foods, and avoiding high-carb foods. It should be at least 70% fat, around 25% protein, and only 5% carbohydrates. When choosing foods, pick those that are closest to their natural forms. As much as possible, choose raw over preserved foods, organic over highly processed, grass-fed or free-range over caged animals, wild caught over farmed fish, etc.

Below is a list of low-carb foods you can choose from:

Fats & oils

- Almond
- Avocado
- Butter
- Ghee
- Lard
- Olive
- Nut oils
- Seed oils
- Mayonnaise
- Peanut butter
- Cocoa butter
- Coconut
- Chicken fat
- Beef tallow
- Bacon fat

Note: Limit intake of oils rich in omega-6 fatty acids, such as nut oil, canola oil, corn oil, sunflower oil and margarine. Choose cold pressed vegetable oils.

Meat

- Beef
- Bacon
- Pork chops
- Lamb
- Veal
- Ham
- Goat
- Pork loin
- Wild game
- Sausage
- Chicken
- Duck
- Quail
- Goose
- Turkey
- Pheasant
- Any wild-caught fish or seafood

- Whole eggs

Note: Choose fattier cuts of meat from grass-fed or free-range animals.

Vegetables

- Asparagus
- Alfalfa
- Avocado
- Bell pepper
- Bamboo sprouts
- Brussels sprouts
- Beet greens
- Broccoli
- Bean sprouts
- Bok choy
- Celery
- Cabbage
- Carrots
- Chives
- Cucumber
- Cauliflower

- Chard
- Collard greens
- Leeks
- Radishes
- Onion
- Kale
- Garlic
- Spinach
- Scallions
- Tomatoes
- Snow peas
- Summer squash
- Shallot
- Water chestnut
- Turnip

Note: Avoid starchy veggies such as potatoes, winter squash, etc.

Nuts & seeds

- Almond
- Macadamia

- Walnut
- Pecan
- Cashew
- Chestnut
- Pistachio
- Any kind of seeds

Note: Nuts and seeds are high in omega-6 fatty acids and some have higher carb content, so it is best to limit intake. They are best consumed when soaked and roasted.

Dairy

- Whipping cream
- Sour cream
- Cream cheese
- Any kind of cheese
- Yogurt

Note: Choose full fat and organic dairy products.

Beverages

- Herbal tea
- Decaf coffee and tea

- Almond milk
- Soy milk
- Coconut milk
- Lime juice
- Lemon juice

Note: Choose unsweetened options.

Sweeteners

- Stevia
- Xylitol
- Monk fruit
- Lo han guo
- Chicory root
- Splenda
- Erythritol

Note: Choose liquid sweeteners over powdered oncs.

Fruits

Berries such as blueberries, strawberries, etc.

Seasonings

Any low-carb spices without added sugar

Benefits of the Ketogenic Diet

Brain protection

The ketogenic diet was originally designed to treat epilepsy, a neurological disease characterized by recurrent and uncontrollable shaking or seizures. These seizures are caused by abnormal and excessive activities of the nerve cells in the brain. Epilepsy is now usually treated with anticonvulsant medications or surgery. But in some cases where such medications are ineffective, a ketogenic diet is implemented.

It is unclear how exactly the diet works, but in many cases it lessens the number of seizures by 50% or more, especially in children. Clinical trials show that ketone bodies have the capacity to protect brain cells from damage and prevent their premature death. They suggest that ketogenic diets can also prevent or reverse other neurodegenerative disorders such as Parkinson's and Alzheimer's. The use of the diet for this purpose is still in the research stage.

Heart health

Many people are skeptical about the ketogenic diet because of its high fat intake. They believe that fats increase cholesterol levels and clog the arteries. However, current studies dismiss this myth and actually prove that a ketogenic diet can be beneficial for the cardiovascular system.

Fats or lipids in the bloodstream can be found in two forms: triglycerides and cholesterol. A triglyceride is a fatty acid that stores energy, and cholesterol is a molecule used by the body to aid in absorption of vitamins, cell maintenance, hormone regulation, etc. This means that fat is essential for the body to function normally. Now, cholesterol is transported throughout the body in the blood by molecules called lipoproteins. These lipoproteins are classified depending on their density: low-density lipoproteins (LDL) and high-density lipoproteins (HDL).

HDL is known as the good cholesterol because it not only transports cholesterol, it also brings unused cholesterol back to the liver to be broken down. This prevents it from clogging the arteries and leading to cardiovascular disease. Thus, increased HDL is ideal for maintaining a healthy cardiovascular system. LDL, on the other hand, is commonly referred to as the bad cholesterol because it moves more slowly than HDL and has a tendency to clog arteries when oxidized by free radicals. LDL comes in different forms: the larger it is the better for you; the smaller and denser the form the more harmful it is.

One study shows that low-carb diets significantly increase the level of HDL cholesterol compared to low-fat diets. Another study suggests that low-carb diets can help reduce LDL levels and increase the size of LDL molecules. The ketogenic diet, therefore, is beneficial to your cardiovascular system as it helps increase the good HDL and decrease the bad LDL.

Weight loss

The most effective way to lose weight permanently is to deal with its root cause. There are many causes of weight gain, but the dominant one is hormonal imbalance. Overeating and living a sedentary lifestyle are obvious reasons for gaining weight; however, these are actually symptoms of a hormonal imbalance related to insulin, the hormone responsible for moving glucose into the cells to be used as fuel. When the body's insulin is abnormally high, it becomes dependent on glucose for fuel and refuses to use up stored fats. This is the underlying reason for overeating. And low energy levels, caused by the hormonal imbalance, hinder a more active lifestyle.

The main cause of increased insulin levels is high carbohydrate consumption, which is a common feature of an average diet. When glucose from carbs accumulates in the blood, the body releases more insulin in order to deal with it. Too much carb intake increases both levels of blood sugar and insulin. This will eventually lead to high blood pressure, weight gain and other related diseases.

In other words, the ketogenic diet is one of the best weight loss programs because it maintains normal levels of insulin, keeps hormones balanced and prevents any increase of blood sugar levels. You will feel fewer cravings, which helps prevent overeating; and you'll have higher energy levels for more activities that help you lose weight.

Summary

The purpose of the ketogenic diet is primarily for health improvement, but because of its weight loss benefits many dieters have joined the program. Fortunately, the keto diet plan is a healthy and easy way to lose those extra pounds. In a keto diet, counting calories is made easy and cooking meals made fun!

Thanks again for downloading this book, I hope you enjoy it!

Ok, onto the recipes...

Enjoy!

BREAKFAST

Almond-Pumpkin Smoothie

Ingredients

2 cups almond milk

1 cup pumpkin puree

1 tsp pure vanilla extract

½ cup water

ice cubes (optional)

cacao nibs (optional)

Instructions

1. Mix all the ingredients in a blender and pulse until silky smooth.

2. Serve in chilled glass and enjoy.

Servings: 3
Cooking Time: 5 minutes

Nutrition Facts

Serving size: 1/3 of a recipe (7.7 ounces)

Percent daily values based on the Reference Daily Intake (RDI) for a 2000 calorie diet.

Amount Per Serving

Calories 285.1

Calories From Fat (85%) 243.1

% Daily Value

Total Fat 29.0g 45%

Saturated Fat 25.7g 129%

Cholesterol 0mg 0%

Sodium 117.4mg 5%

Potassium 384.9mg 11%

Total Carbohydrates 7.3g 2%

Fiber 1.2g 5%

Sugar 1.5g

Protein 3.2g 6%

Curly Kale "Ice Cream" Shake

Ingredients

1 ½ cup curly green kale leaves

½ cup heavy (whipping) cream

½ cup filtered water

½ cup raw cashews

2 Tbsp liquid sweetener of your choice

1 tsp vanilla extract

1 tsp finely minced ginger

pinch of Celtic sea salt

ice cubes (optional)

Instructions

1. Throw all of the ingredients in your blender and puree until smooth and creamy. 2. Add ice cubes and enjoy your day!

Servings: 2

Preparation: 5 minutes

Nutrition Facts

Serving size: 1/2 of a recipe (7.7 ounces)

Percent daily values based on the Reference Daily Intake (RDI) for a 2000 calorie diet.

Amount Per Serving

Calories 141.2

Calories From Fat (50%) 69.9

% Daily Value

Total Fat 8.4g 13%

Saturated Fat 1.6g 8%

Cholesterol 0mg 0%

Sodium 28.6mg 1%

Potassium 390.2mg 11%

Total Carbohydrates 9.2g 3%

Fiber 2g 8%

Sugar 2.7g

Protein 4.5g 9%

Easy Lemon Poppy Seed Muffins

Ingredients

4 eggs

2 tsp poppy seeds

1 tsp sesame seeds

1 cup almond flour

4 Tbsp olive oil

½ cup sweetener of your choice

3 Tbsp lemon juice

1 tsp vanilla extract

½ tsp baking soda

zest of one lemon

salt

Instructions

1. Preheat oven to 320°F. Prepare 12 muffin cups.

2. Place all ingredients in your blender and mix well until smooth.

3. Divide batter evenly among the muffin cups. Bake for 30 minutes.

4. When ready, cool and serve.

Servings: 12

Cooking Time

Total Time: 40 minutes

Nutrition Facts

Serving size: 1/12 of a recipe (1.3 ounces)

Percent daily values based on the Reference Daily Intake (RDI) for a 2000 calorie diet.

Amount Per Serving

Calories 111.2

Calories From Fat (52%) 57.3

% Daily Value

Total Fat 6.5g 10%

Saturated Fat 4.7g 24%

Cholesterol 47.1mg 16%

Sodium 71.4mg 3%

Potassium 49.7mg 1%

Total Carbohydrates 8.4g 2%

Fiber 0.5g 2%

Sugar 2.7g

Protein 2.9g 6%

Homemade Energetic Bar

Ingredients

1 cup almonds

¼ cup pecans

1 cup peanuts

1 cup shredded coconut

1 cup almond butter

1 cup coconut oil, freshly melted and still warm

4 Tbsp sweetener of your choice (optional)

1 Tbsp chocolate chips (optional)

Instructions

1. Place the almonds, pecans, peanuts in a food processor and chop them for 1 to 2 minutes.

2. Add in the shredded coconut, almond butter, sweetener and coconut oil. Process for one minute.

3. Place parchment paper on a square container and place the mixture on top.

4. Whisk the mixture vigorously, with a spatula and then with the hand.

5. Place the chocolate chips on top and press them slightly with your hands.

6. Place the container in the freezer for 3 to 4 hours.

7. Remove from the freezer and cut into rectangular pieces with a large knife.

8. Serve.

Servings: 8

Nutrition Facts

Serving size: 1/8 of a recipe (1.3 ounces)

Amount Per Serving

Calories 223.4

Calories From Fat (78%) 174.6

% Daily Value

Total Fat 20.7g 32%

Saturated Fat 8.6g 43%

Cholesterol 0mg 0%

Sodium 32.4mg 1%

Potassium 163.5mg 5%

Total Carbohydrates 8.2g 3%

Fiber 2.8g 11%

Sugar 3.3g

Protein 4.5g 9%

Mediterranean Mint and Feta Omelette

Ingredients

3 eggs

6 fresh mint leaves

4 ounces feta cheese

salt and freshly ground black pepper, to taste

olive oil

Instructions

1. In bowl, beat eggs with feta cheese and chopped fresh mint. Season salt and pepper. Mix well.

2. In a frying pan add olive oil and pour the egg mixture; cook over medium to high heat for 2 to 3 minutes.

3. With the wooden spoon turn the omelette to other side and cook one minute more.

4. When done, the bottom will be set and the edges will look crisp.

5. Transfer omelette to a plate and serve hot. Enjoy!

Servings: 2

Cooking Time

Total Time: 15 minutes

Nutrition Facts

Serving size: 1/2 of a recipe (2.8 ounces)

Percent daily values based on the Reference Daily Intake (RDI) for a 2000 calorie diet.

Amount Per Serving

Calories 113.7

Calories From Fat (60%) 68.1

% Daily Value

Total Fat 7.6g 12%

Saturated Fat 2.6g 13%

Cholesterol 279.9mg 93%

Sodium 259.7mg 11%

Potassium 113.2mg 3%

Total Carbohydrates 0.8g <1%

Fiber 0.1g <1%

Sugar 0.3g

Protein 9.9g 20%

Nutty Eggs with Avocado

Ingredients

4 large eggs

½ avocado, sliced

½ cup walnuts, sliced

2 Tbsp olive oil

½ tsp cilantro (optional)

sea salt and freshly ground black pepper to taste

Instructions

1. Heat the oil in a skillet over medium-high heat.

2. Beat the eggs in a small bowl and pour into the skillet.

3. Cook for 1 minute and turn heat to medium-low. Cook about 3 minutes more.

4. Top with walnuts, avocado and cilantro.

5. Season with sea salt and freshly ground black pepper to taste.

6. Serve.

Servings: 2

Nutrition Facts

Serving size: 1/2 of a recipe (5.1 ounces)

Percent daily values based on the Reference Daily Intake (RDI) for a 2000 calorie diet.

Amount Per Serving

Calories 286.5

Calories From Fat (73%) 208.8

% Daily Value

Total Fat 24.5g 38%

Saturated Fat 4.1g 20%

Cholesterol 247.4mg 82%

Sodium 194.5mg 8%

Potassium 438mg 13%

Total Carbohydrates 7.6g 3%

Fiber 4.4g 18%

Sugar 1.3g

Protein 2.1g 24%

Pancake Torte with Ham and Bacon

Ingredients

6 keto pancakes

4 slices of bacon

4 slices ham

2 cups shredded cheddar cheese

fresh parsley (chopped)

coconut oil

Instructions

1. Top one keto pancake with one slice of bacon, ham, parsley and shredded cheese.

2. Place another pancake on top of the filling and repeat the procedure.

3. Continue until you finish with all bacon, ham and cheese.

4. Cook in frying pan on medium-low heat with coconut oil, and cover with a lid until the cheese is melted.

5. Flip and cook 1-2 minutes on the other side.

6. Let cool. Cut and serve hot.

Servings: 8

Cooking Time

Preparation Time: 25 minutes

Nutrition Facts

Serving size: 1/8 of a recipe (3.5 ounces)

Percent daily values based on the Reference Daily Intake (RDI) for a 2000 calorie diet.

Amount Per Serving

Calories 314.1

Calories From Fat (66%) 207.7

% Daily Value

Total Fat 23.3g 36%

Saturated Fat 10.8g 54%

Cholesterol 74.7mg 25%

Sodium 737.1mg 31%

Potassium 168.7mg 5%

Total Carbohydrates 8.6g 3%

Fiber 0g 0%

Sugar 0.2g

Protein 16.9g 34%

Vegetable Omelette

Ingredients

3 eggs

1 medium zucchini

1 green onion (white and green parts), chopped

1 green pepper

2 tsp parmesan cheese – grated

2 cloves garlic

Salt and ground black pepper to taste

Instructions

1. Wash and dry all vegetables and dice finely.

2. Heat frying pan with the olive oil and sauté the garlic, green onion and pepper about 5 minutes. Add salt and pepper to taste.

3. Add the diced zucchini, stir and cook 3-4 minutes more.

4. In a bowl, beat the eggs with parmesan cheese.

5. Pour egg mixture over the vegetables and cook for 3 minutes per side.

6. Serve hot.

Servings: 3

Cooking Time

Total Time: 35 minutes

Nutrition Facts

Serving size: 1/3 of a recipe (10.6 ounces)

Percent daily values based on the Reference Daily Intake (RDI) for a 2000 calorie diet.

Amount Per Serving

Calories 128.4

Calories From Fat (37%) 47.4

% Daily Value

Total Fat 5.3g 8%

Saturated Fat 1.7g 8%

Cholesterol 186mg 62%

Sodium 84.4mg 4%

Potassium 614.2mg 18%

Total Carbohydrates 9.7g 4%

Fiber 3.3g 13%

Sugar 7.2g

Protein 8.9g 18%

LUNCH

Baked Pickled Cabbage with Ham

Ingredients

14 oz ham

3 green onions, chopped

2 bay leaves

1 head pickled cabbage

4 cloves garlic (chopped)

2 dry red peppers

a few peppercorns

4 Tbsp oil

salt & black pepper to taste

Instructions

1. Preheat oven to 400°F.

2. Cut the ham into pieces and put in a saucepan with water; bring to boil.

3. Add the onion (cut in half or in quarters), bay leaf and a few peppercorns.

4. Cook about 30 minutes.

5. Remove the ham and set aside on a plate.

6. Chop the onion, leek and dry red paprika.

7. In a separate bowl, finely chop the pickled cabbage.

8. Heat the large frying pan with oil, add the onion and chopped dried peppers, and stir well.

9. Add the cabbage and cook about 30 minutes over medium heat, stirring constantly. Adjust salt and ground black pepper to taste. Remove from the fire.

10. In a greased baking dish put half of the fried cabbage, layer with the ham, and cover with the remaining cabbage.

11. Pour just enough water to cover the cabbage.

12. Bake in the oven for about 1 hour. Serve hot.

Servings: 8

Cooking Time

Total Time: 2 hours

Nutrition Facts

Serving size: 1/8 of a recipe (9 ounces).

Percent daily values based on the Reference Daily Intake (RDI) for a 2000 calorie diet.

Amount Per Serving

Calories 174.5

Calories From Fat (42%) 72.9

% Daily Value

Total Fat 8.2g 13%

Saturated Fat 1.6g 8%

Cholesterol 11mg 4%

Sodium 480.6mg 20%

Potassium 437.7mg 13%

Total Carbohydrates 15.7g 5%

Fiber 4.8g 19%

Sugar 6.8g

Protein 11.5g 23%

Beef, Asparagus and Mushroom Stew

Ingredients

1 ¼ lb beef filets

½ lb mushrooms, thinly sliced

1 cup asparagus, cooked and cut into small pieces

2 cloves garlic

2 green onions, finely chopped

½ cup bell pepper (green or red)

1 tsp minced garlic

pinch of turmeric

2 Tbsp olive oil

½ tsp dried rosemary

Salt and freshly ground black pepper to taste

Instructions

1. Add the oil in an oven-proof skillet. Add in the onion, red pepper, and garlic and sauté 2-3 minutes.

2. Add mushrooms and cook for two to three minutes more. Stir in rosemary, salt and pepper to taste.

3. In medium bowl, combine the onion mixture with asparagus and beef chunks and set aside.

4. In a greased frying skillet over medium-high heat, cook meat and the vegetable mixture.

5. Reduce heat to medium-low and cook 10 to 15 minutes.

6. Serve hot.

Servings: 6

Cooking Time

Total Time: 35 minutes

Nutrition Facts

Serving size: 1/6 of a recipe (7.5 ounces)

Percent daily values based on the Reference Daily Intake (RDI) for a 2000 calorie diet.

Amount Per Serving

Calories 315.4

Calories From Fat (71%) 222.5

% Daily Value

Total Fat 24.3g 37%

Saturated Fat 8.5g 43%

Cholesterol 70.9mg 24%

Sodium 69.9mg 3%

Potassium 521.2mg 15%

Total Carbohydrates 5g 2%

Fiber 1.9g 8%

Sugar 2.3g

Protein 19.3g 39%

Cashews Chicken and Watercress Stir-Fry

Ingredients

1 ¼ lb beef filets

½ lb mushrooms, thinly sliced

1 cup asparagus, cooked and cut into small pieces

2 cloves garlic

2 green onions, finely chopped

½ cup bell pepper (green or red)

1 tsp minced garlic

pinch of turmeric

2 Tbsp olive oil

½ tsp dried rosemary

Salt and freshly ground black pepper to taste

Instructions

1. Add the oil in an oven-proof skillet. Add in the onion, red pepper, and garlic and sauté 2-3 minutes.

2. Add mushrooms and cook for two to three minutes more. Stir in rosemary, salt and pepper to taste.

3. In medium bowl, combine the onion mixture with asparagus and beef chunks and set aside.

4. In a greased frying skillet over medium-high heat, cook meat and the vegetable mixture.

5. Reduce heat to medium-low and cook 10 to 15 minutes.

6. Serve hot.

Servings: 6

Cooking Time

Total Time: 35 minutes

Nutrition Facts

Serving size: 1/6 of a recipe (7.5 ounces)

Percent daily values based on the Reference Daily Intake (RDI) for a 2000 calorie diet.

Amount Per Serving

Calories 315.4

Calories From Fat (71%) 222.5

% Daily Value

Total Fat 24.3g 37%

Saturated Fat 8.5g 43%

Cholesterol 70.9mg 24%

Sodium 69.9mg 3%

Potassium 521.2mg 15%

Total Carbohydrates 5g 2%

Fiber 1.9g 8%

Sugar 2.3g

Protein 19.3g 39%

Creamy Zucchini and Broccoli Soup

Ingredients

2 leeks (white part only)

4 big green zucchinis

1 cup broccoli (shredded)

3 Tbsp virgin olive oil

5 cups water

Salt and black pepper, to taste

Parmesan cheese – grated

Instructions

1. Heat the olive oil in a large saucepan, and add the chopped leeks.

2. Cook the leeks until soft (8-10 minutes), stirring gently.

3. Add the chopped zucchini and broccoli and sauté about 5 minutes.

4. Add water, bring to a boil and simmer without covering for about 15-17 minutes.

5. Process the soup in batches until smooth.

6. Ladle to plates, sprinkle with grated cheese and serve.

Servings: 4

Cooking Time

Total Time: 45 minutes

Nutrition Facts

Serving size: 1/4 of a recipe (15.7 ounces).

Percent daily values based on the Reference Daily Intake (RDI) for a 2000 calorie diet.

Amount Per Serving

Calories 74.9

Calories From Fat (9%) 6.6

% Daily Value

Total Fat 0.8g 1%

Saturated Fat 0.2g <1%

Cholesterol 0mg 0%

Sodium 176.4mg 7%

Potassium 672.4mg 19%

Total Carbohydrates 11.7g 5%

Fiber 3.2g 13%

Sugar 5.0g

Protein 3.4g 7%

Curry Broccoli Cream Soup

Ingredients

1 ¼ lb broccoli

1 cup cauliflower florets

2 green onions (green parts only, minced)

2 white celery stalks

3 Tbsp olive oil

1 onion

3 cups water

curry to taste

ginger

salt and pepper (to taste)

splash of cream or evaporated milk

Instructions

1. In a saucepan or pot with oil, sauté chopped green onion and celery.

2. Add in the broccoli and cauliflower.

3. Add the curry, ground ginger and salt and pepper to taste.

4. Pour in water to cover the vegetables. Bring to boil and cook 10-12 minutes over low heat.

5. Once everything is cooked through, place in a blender, add a splash of cream or evaporated milk, and blend until smooth.

6. Adjust salt to taste and serve.

Servings: 4

Cooking Time

Total Time: 40 minutes

Nutrition Facts

Serving size: 1/4 of a recipe (10.9 ounces)

Percent daily values based on the Reference Daily Intake (RDI) for a 2000 calorie diet.

Amount Per Serving

Calories 164.4

Calories From Fat (56%) 91.2

% Daily Value

Total Fat 10.3g 16%

Saturated Fat 1.4g 7%

Cholesterol 0mg 0%

Sodium 18.5mg <1%

Potassium 321.3mg 9%

Total Carbohydrates 11.2g 6%

Fiber 2.3g 9%

Sugar 3.4g

Protein 1.9g 4%

Keto Grilled Shrimps

Ingredients

14 ounces fresh shrimp

2 Tbsp olive oil

sea-salt flakes

rosemary sprig, leaves finely chopped

Instructions

1. Rinse the whole shrimp and then drain them.

2. Heat some oil on a grill pan. Place shrimp on grill and cook 5-7 minutes, turning halfway through the process.

3. The outside of the shrimp should turn a nice pink color when it is cooked.

4. Place shrimp on the serving plate and sprinkle with sea-salt flakes.

5. Serve.

Servings: 2

Cooking Time

Total Time: 30 minutes

Nutrition Facts

Serving size: 1/2 of a recipe (7.6 ounces)

Percent daily values based on the Reference Daily Intake (RDI) for a 2000 calorie diet.

Amount Per Serving

Calories 119.3

Calories From Fat (91%) 101.3

% Daily Value

Total Fat 13.5g 21%

Saturated Fat 1.9g 9%

Cholesterol 0mg 0%

Sodium 0.3mg <1%

Potassium 0.1mg <1%

Total Carbohydrates 0g 0%

Fiber 0g 0%

Sugar 0g

Protein 0g 0%

Lemony Grilled Chicken

Ingredients

3 lbs chicken breast

5 limes or lemons, sliced

1 tsp allspice

1 Tbsp onion powder

1 Tbsp smoked paprika

1 Tbsp garlic powder

sea salt and freshly ground black pepper to taste

Instructions

1. Prepare your barbecue grill.

2. In a large bowl, place chicken pieces and lemon rings.

3. In a small bowl, combine paprika, onion powder, garlic powder, allspice, salt and pepper to taste.

4. Pour the spice mixture over chicken and mix thoroughly.

5. Grill chicken and lemon rings on barbecue over medium heat for 10-12 minutes per side.

6. Sprinkle with chopped parsley and serve hot.

Servings: 6

Cooking Time

Total Time: 45 minutes

Nutrition Facts

Serving size: 1/6 of a recipe (11.3 ounces)

Percent daily values based on the Reference Daily Intake (RDI) for a 2000 calorie diet.

Amount Per Serving

Calories 289.9

Calories From Fat (19%) 55.6

% Daily Value

Total Fat 6.3g 10%

Saturated Fat 1.4g 7%

Cholesterol 145.2mg 48%

Sodium 268.6mg 11%

Potassium 1029.4mg 29%

Total Carbohydrates 9.6g 4%

Fiber 5.0g 20%

Sugar 0.2g

Protein 29.8g 50%

Mackerel Fish and Shrimp Soup (Slow Cooker)

Ingredients

1 lb mackerel fish fillets

2 cups frozen shrimp

1 cup cauliflower florets

½ cup carrots

1 cup zucchini (medium, sliced)

½ green onion finely chopped

heart of celery

2 cloves garlic

1 cup heavy whipping cream

3 cups water

salt and fresh ground pepper to taste

Instructions

1. Chop up the vegetables.

2. Cube the fish and dump everything (except the cream and the shrimp) into your slow cooker.

3. Cover and cook on LOW for 8-10 hours.

4. About 30 minutes before serving, stir in your cup of cream and the frozen shrimp.

5. Turn your slow cooker to HIGH for the last 30 minutes.

6. Serve hot.

Servings: 6

Cooking Time

Total Time: 9 hours

Nutrition Facts

Serving size: 1/6 of a recipe (9.3 ounces)

Percent daily values based on the Reference Daily Intake (RDI) for a 2000 calorie diet.

Amount Per Serving

Calories 235.3

Calories From Fat (63%) 147.8

% Daily Value

Total Fat 16.8g 26%

Saturated Fat 9.7g 48%

Cholesterol 84.9mg 28%

Sodium 288mg 12%

Potassium 266.9mg 8%

Total Carbohydrates 3.7g 1%

Fiber 0.6g 2%

Sugar 0.9g

Protein 17.4g 35%

Savory Belgian Endives Salad with Cheddar

Ingredients

4 Belgian endives

2 oz cheddar cheese, cut into small cubes

3 Tbsp fresh parsley leaves, coarsely chopped

3 Tbsp fresh lemon juice

3 Tbsp of olive oil

Salt and pepper to taste

Instructions

1. Cut and remove the bottom of the endives and wash in cold water.

2. In a bowl, whisk well the olive oil, lemon juice and salt and pepper to taste.

3. Place endives in a salad bowl and add the cheddar cheese cubes and the chopped parsley.

4. Sprinkle with lemon juice dressing, toss the salad, and serve immediately.

Servings: 4

Cooking Time

Total Time: 15 minutes

Nutrition Facts

Serving size: 1/4 of a recipe (6.9 ounces)

Percent daily values based on the Reference Daily Intake (RDI) for a 2000 calorie diet.

Amount Per Serving

Calories 150.2

Calories From Fat (87%) 131.3

% Daily Value

Total Fat 14.9g 23%

Saturated Fat 4.4g 22%

Cholesterol 14.9mg 5%

Sodium 89.9mg 4%

Potassium 41.6mg 1%

Total Carbohydrates 1.2g <1%

Fiber 0.13g <1%

Sugar 0.4g

Protein 3.7g 7%

DINNER

Avocados Stuffed with Shrimp

Ingredients

2 cups small shrimp, cooked and washed

4 large avocados

1 Tbsp lemon juice

2 Tbsp fresh cilantro

2 Tbsp mayonnaise

1 Tbsp onion powder

1 tsp black pepper

1 Tbsp paprika

Salt to taste

Instructions

1. Put the avocados on a plate with the cut side up.

2. In a medium bowl, mix the shrimp, lemon juice, fresh cilantro, onion and pepper. Place the shrimp mixture in each avocado, covering generously.

3. Pour the mayonnaise over stuffed avocados. Serve immediately.

Servings: 6

Nutrition Facts

Serving size: 1/6 of a recipe (5.6 ounces)

Percent daily values based on the Reference Daily Intake (RDI) for a 2000 calorie diet.

Amount Per Serving

Calories 222.1

Calories From Fat (74%) 165.2

% Daily Value

Total Fat 19.6g 30%

Saturated Fat 2.7g 14%

Cholesterol 3.8mg 1%

Sodium 57-96mg 2%

Potassium 640.0mg 18%

Total Carbohydrates 10.1g 4%

Fiber 8.6g 34%

Sugar 0.9g

Protein 2.9g 6%

Chilled Cauliflower and Cilantro Soup

Ingredients

1 lb cauliflower

½ can (11 oz) coconut milk

½ cup water

½ tsp fresh ginger

3 sprigs fresh cilantro

2 Tbsp olive oil

Salt and pepper to taste

Instructions

1. Place the cauliflower in a large pot and cover with water.

2. Bring to a boil over high heat, then reduce heat to medium-low, cover, and simmer 5 to 7 minutes.

3. Remove from heat, drain and let cool several minutes.

4. Put the cauliflower in a bowl and beat together with the coconut milk.

5. While beating, add the water little by little until you get the desired texture.

6. With a mortar, crush the ginger and cilantro and add to the cauliflower.

7. Beat again to combine all the ingredients.

8. Serve cold.

Servings: 4

Nutrition Facts

Serving size: 1/4 of a recipe (4.4 ounces).

Percent daily values based on the Reference Daily Intake (RDI) for a 2000 calorie diet.

Amount Per Serving

Calories 120.8

Calories From Fat (93%) 111.9

% Daily Value

Total Fat 13g 20%

Saturated Fat 6.5g 32%

Cholesterol 0mg 0%

Sodium 5.4mg <1%

Potassium 77.9mg 2%

Total Carbohydrates 1.8g <1%

Fiber 0.0g <1%

Sugar 0.0g

Protein 0.5g 1%

Ground Beef and Kale Stew with Cashews

Ingredients

1 Tbsp coconut oil

1 lb ground beef

2 cups curly kale

1 tsp ground cumin

1 tsp oregano

1 tsp garlic powder

salt and freshly ground black pepper, to taste

1 cup cashews

Instructions

1. In a pan, melt the coconut oil and cook the beef over medium heat.

2. Browning ground beef should take approximately 7 to 10 minutes for 1 pound of meat.

3. Add the cumin, oregano, garlic powder, ground pepper and salt; stir.

4. Add chopped kale and cook for 5 minutes.

5. Remove from the heat, sprinkle with chopped cashews and serve.

Servings: 4

Nutrition Facts

Serving size: 1/4 of a recipe (7.2 ounces)

Percent daily values based on the Reference Daily Intake (RDI) for a 2000 calorie diet.

Amount Per Serving

Calories 397.6

Calories From Fat (74%) 412.5

% Daily Value

Total Fat 35.8g 59%

Saturated Fat 19.6g 98%

Cholesterol 150mg 50%

Sodium 138.8mg 6%

Potassium 536.0mg 15%

Total Carbohydrates 0.7g <1%

Fiber 0.2g <1%

Sugar 0.0g

Protein 35.5g 71%

Kale Broccoli Cream Soup

Ingredients

1 ¾ lb broccoli

2 scalions, chopped

2 celery stalks, chopped

1 ½ cups kale (finely chopped)

ginger

curry to taste

3 Tbsp olive oil (or butter)

water

Instructions

1. Heat the oil in a pot; sauté chopped green onion and celery 1 to 2 minutes.

2. Add in the broccoli and kale. Add salt and pepper to taste, and add in the curry and ground ginger.

3. Pour water to cover vegetables, cover and boil for 4 to 5 minutes, until tender.

4. Once everything is cooked through, beat until a very thin consistency is reached and add a splash of cream or evaporated milk.

5. Adjust salt and pepper and serve.

Servings: 4

Cooking Time

Total Time: 40 minutes

Nutrition Facts

Serving size: 1/4 of a recipe (7.2 ounces).

Percent daily values based on the Reference Daily Intake (RDI) for a 2000 calorie diet.

Amount Per Serving

Calories 173.5

Calories From Fat (53%) 91.5

% Daily Value

Total Fat 10.4g 16%

Saturated Fat 1.4g 7%

Cholesterol 0mg 0%

Sodium 31.4mg 1%

Potassium 430.6mg 12%

Total Carbohydrates 11.0g 4%

Fiber 2.7g 11%

Sugar 2.7g

Protein 2.2g 4%

Salmon Ratatouille

Ingredients

1 lb salmon

1 scallion, roughly chopped

1 green pepper

1 eggplant

1 zucchini

3 Tbsp extra virgin olive oil

½ cup water

1 tsp sweet pepper powder

pepper & salt to taste

dill

granulated garlic

Instructions

1. Preheat oven to 400°F.

2. In a frying pan with olive oil, sauté chopped eggplant and zucchini 3 to 4 minutes.

3. Add in chopped scallion and green pepper.

4. Cover; cook over medium-low heat, stirring often, for 7 to 10 minutes, or until eggplant is tender.

5. Pour the water, cover and cook for an additional 20 minutes.

6. Add in one teaspoon of sweet pepper powder. Adjust salt and pepper.

7. Spread the aluminium paper over your working surface. Share the vegetable mixture among three or four aluminium pieces.

8. Place the salmon over the vegetables and close the wrap.

9. Place the salmon wraps in the oven and bake for 15-17 minutes.

10. Serve hot.

Servings: 4

Cooking Time

Total Time: 55 minutes

Nutrition Facts

Serving size: 1/4 of a recipe (9.3 ounces).

Percent daily values based on the Reference Daily Intake (RDI) for a 2000 calorie diet.

Amount Per Serving

Calories 80.2

Calories From Fat (5%) 4.1

% Daily Value

Total Fat 0.5g <1%

Saturated Fat 0.1g <1%

Cholesterol 0.1mg <1%

Sodium 15.2mg <1%

Potassium 527.5mg 15%

Total Carbohydrates 9.4g 4%

Fiber 5.6g 22%

Sugar 5.4g

Protein 2.5g 5%

Slow Cooker Beef Soup

Ingredients

1 ½ lbs round steak

1 cup scallion, roughly chopped

2 cups water

1 cup sweet potato, peeled and cut into cubes

1 carrot, sliced thinly

4 Tbsp lemon juice

salt and pepper, to taste

2 Tbsp olive oil

Instructions

1. Add beef strips to the bottom of your slow cooker.

2. Add the oil, chopped scallions, carrots and sweet potato.

3. Pour in water, cover and cook on LOW 6 to 8 hours.

4. Serve hot.

Servings: 6

Cooking Time

Total Time: 8 hours

Nutrition Facts

Serving size: 1/6 of a recipe (9.1 ounces)

Percent daily values based on the Reference Daily Intake (RDI) for a 2000 calorie diet.

Amount Per Serving

Calories 282.4

Calories From Fat (59%) 167.1

% Daily Value

Total Fat 18.6g 29%

Saturated Fat 5.6g 28%

Cholesterol 70.3mg 23%

Sodium 95.6mg 4%

Potassium 534.1mg 15%

Total Carbohydrates 7.6g 3%

Fiber 1.5g 6%

Sugar 2.2g

Protein 20.6g 41%

Spinach Almond Purée

Ingredients

1 lb fresh spinach (well washed)

2 cups cauliflower florets

2 green onions (white and green parts), chopped

4 Tbsp olive oil

4 cups water

¼ cup roasted almonds, chopped

Instructions

1. Wash, clean and cut all vegetables.

2. In a non-stick frying pan, fry the almonds 2-3 minutes; remove from the heat and set aside.

3. Heat the olive oil in a deep pan and cook the cauliflower and green onion for about two minutes.

4. Add the cleaned spinach leaves, water and salt to taste. Bring to a boil and let it simmer for 15 minutes.

5. Remove from the heat and place the vegetables in a food processor along with some toasted almonds. Blend until smooth.

6. Ladle purée into bowls and serve.

Servings: 4

Cooking Time

Total Time: 45 minutes

Nutrition Facts

Serving size: 1/4 of a recipe (13.4 ounces)

Amount Per Serving

Calories 72.4

Calories From Fat (36%) 26.0

% Daily Value

Total Fat 3.1g 5%

Saturated Fat 0.3g 2%

Cholesterol 0mg 0%

Sodium 122.2mg 5%

Potassium 906.1mg 26%

Total Carbohydrates 8.7g 3%

Fiber 4.6g 18%

Sugar 1.9g

Protein 5.7g 11%

Stuffed Portobello Mushrooms

Ingredients

8 large Portobello mushrooms

2 leeks

1 spring onion (medium-large)

1 green pepper

2 Tbsp cream

4 Tbsp parmesan cheese

salt and pepper to taste

Instructions

1. Preheat oven to 350°F.

2. Clean the mushrooms with a damp paper towel. Remove the stems and cut in half.

3. Cut the green and hard part of the leeks. Cut in half lengthwise and wash

4. well under a stream of water, opening the leaves to remove any dirt. Cut into thin slices.

5. Wash and remove the stalks and white parts of the peppers; chop into cubes.

6. In a large skillet heat 1 tablespoon vegetable oil or butter over medium heat and cook the leeks, stirring about 5 minutes.

7. Add the chopped vegetables and cook about 3-4 more minutes, stirring occasionally. Season with salt and pepper to taste.

8. Add the cream and turn off the heat; stir until incorporated well.

9. Place the mushrooms in a greased baking pan and season with salt.

10. Stuff every mushroom with the vegetable mixture and sprinkle with parmesan cheese.

11. Bake in oven for 25 minutes.

12. Serve hot.

Servings: 8

Cooking Time

Total Time: 55 minutes

Nutrition Facts

Serving size: 1/8 of a recipe (7.5 ounces)

Percent daily values based on the Reference Daily Intake (RDI) for a 2000 calorie diet.

Amount Per Serving

Calories 85.2

Calories From Fat (30%) 25.2

% Daily Value

Total Fat 2.9g 4%

Saturated Fat 1.5g 7%

Cholesterol 7.0mg 2%

Sodium 116.9mg 5%

Potassium 675.0mg 19%

Total Carbohydrates 10.8g 4%

Fiber 2.9g 11%

Sugar 4.4g

Protein 6.4g 13%

Sweet Potato and Spinach Tortilla

Ingredients

1 ¼ cup grated sweet potato

6 eggs (preferably organic)

2 cups spinach

1 Tbsp olive oil

1 green onion, diced

2 Tbsp minced parsley

salt to taste

Instructions

1. In a large bowl beat the eggs and combine with chopped parsley. Set aside.

2. Heat the olive oil in a frying pan and sauté the onion and the sweet potatoes.

3. Season with salt; cook over medium heat for 5 minutes, stirring occasionally.

4. Add the spinach and cook for another 1 minute.

5. Add this mixture to the eggs and mix well.

6. Pour the egg and spinach mixture in the pan and cook for 3 minutes per side over medium heat.

7. Serve hot.

Servings: 4

Cooking Time

Total Time: 30 minutes

Nutrition Facts

Serving size: 1/4 of a recipe (7.7 ounces)

Percent daily values based on the Reference Daily Intake (RDI) for a 2000 calorie diet.

Amount Per Serving

Calories 138.5

Calories From Fat (58%) 80.0

% Daily Value

Total Fat 8.9g 14%

Saturated Fat 2.6g 13%

Cholesterol 279mg 93%

Sodium 193.3mg 8%

Potassium 242.4mg 7%

Total Carbohydrates 4.1g 1%

Fiber 0.9g 4%

Sugar 1.7g

Protein 10.2g 20%

SNACKS

Absolute Avocado Pizza

Ingredients

dough

2 eggs

4 Tbsp grated cheese

2 envelopes unflavored gelatin

1/2 cup sour cream

4 Tbsp water

3 Tbsp butter

salt to taste

fresh parsley (chopped)

filling: ham, bacon, cheddar / mozzarella cheese, mushrooms, avocado puree (instead of tomato sauce)

Instructions

1. Preheat oven to 450°F.

2. Place all ingredients in a blender (without dissolving the gelatin) and beat well.

3. Grease parchment paper with butter and evenly distribute the dough.

5. Place in greased baking pan and bake about 15 minutes.

6. Remove pizza from the oven and spread evenly with avocado sauce.

7. Top with ham, bacon, fresh parsley and mushrooms and sprinkle with the cheese.

8. Bake for 5-10 minutes.

9. Remove from oven, slice and serve immediately.

Servings: 4

Cooking Time
Total Time: 30 minutes

Nutrition Facts
Serving size: 1/4 of a recipe (5.7 ounces)

Percent daily values based on the Reference Daily Intake (RDI) for a 2000 calorie diet.

Amount Per Serving
Calories 267.7

Calories From Fat (69%) 184.6

% Daily Value

Total Fat 20.87g 32%

Saturated Fat 11.4g 57%

Cholesterol 162.8mg 54%

Sodium 800.1mg 33%

Potassium 242.0mg 7%

Total Carbohydrates 1.2g <1%

Fiber 0g 0%

Sugar 0.2g

Protein 18.3g 37%

Baked Parsnip Fingers

Ingredients

2 parsnips, sliced

2 Tbsp olive oil

salt to taste

Instructions

1. Preheat oven to 350°F.

2. Wash, peel and cut the parsnip in sticks. Season with salt to taste.

3. Line a baking pan with parchment paper and toss olive oil over it.

5. Place in oven and bake about 10-12 minutes until golden brown.

6. Serve hot or cold.

Servings: 6

Cooking Time

Total Time: 20 minutes

Nutrition Facts

Serving size: 1/6 of a recipe (3.3 ounces)

Percent daily values based on the Reference Daily Intake (RDI) for a 2000 calorie diet.

Amount Per Serving

Calories 106.5

Calories From Fat (39%) 42.0

% Daily Value

Total Fat 4.8g 7%

Saturated Fat 0.7g 3%

Cholesterol 0mg 0%

Sodium 9.0mg <1%

Potassium 333.8mg 10%

Total Carbohydrates 10.0g 4%

Fiber 4.4g 17%

Sugar 4.3g

Protein 1.1g 2%

Flaxee Eggplant Dip

Ingredients

3 medium eggplants, peeled

6 Tbsp flaxseed flour

1 Tbsp extra virgin olive oil

2 cloves garlic

1 green onion, chopped

1 cup light mayonnaise

salt to taste

water

Instructions

1. Place eggplant, chopped green onion, garlic, water and salt in a pot and bring to a boil.

2. Cover and cook over medium heat for 12-13 minutes, or until eggplant cubes are cooked and soft.

3. Drain in a strainer and allow to cool.

4. Remove from heat and add flaxseed meal. Add the mayonnaise until a smooth paste forms.

5. Serve with your favorite keto crackers.

Servings: 8

Cooking Time

Total Time: 25 minutes

Nutrition Facts

Serving size: 1/8 of a recipe (3.4 ounces)

Percent daily values based on the Reference Daily Intake (RDI) for a 2000 calorie diet.

Amount Per Serving

Calories 122.4

Calories From Fat (85%) 104.3

% Daily Value

Total Fat 11.6g 18%

Saturated Fat 1.7g 9%

Cholesterol 10.5mg 4%

Sodium 240.0mg 10%

Potassium 40.9mg 1%

Total Carbohydrates 4.2g 1%

Fiber 0.3g 1%

Sugar 1.9g

Protein 0.4g <1%

Italiano Fat Balls

Ingredients

1 cup cream cheese

7 slices bacon

¼ cup green olives, pitted and chopped

2 Tbsp fresh basil, chopped

2 Tbsp pesto sauce

1 tsp fresh parsley, chopped

salt and pepper to taste

Instructions

1. Slice pitted olives and the bacon into small pieces.

2. In a bowl, mix together cream cheese, basil and pesto.

3. Add the olives and bacon into the cream cheese and mix again. Add fresh parsley. Mix well.

4. Form into 6 balls and serve immediately.

5. Keep refrigerated

Servings: 6

Cooking Time

Total Time: 10 minutes

Nutrition Facts

Serving size: 1/6 of a recipe (3.4 ounces)

Percent daily values based on the Reference Daily Intake (RDI) for a 2000 calorie diet.

Amount Per Serving

Calories 370.6

Calories From Fat (87%) 322.5

% Daily Value

Total Fat 36.2g 56%

Saturated Fat 14.8g 74%

Cholesterol 74.1mg 25%

Sodium 577.8mg 24%

Potassium 203.5mg 6%

Total Carbohydrates 3.3g 1%

Fiber 0.8g 3%

Sugar 1.3g

Protein 8.7g 17%

Peppermint Artichoke Hearts

Ingredients

6 artichoke hearts with stems, row trimmed

4 cloves garlic, minced

3 cups water

4 Tbsp extra-virgin olive oil

3 Tbsp fresh peppermint leaves, chopped

3 Tbsp fresh cilantro leaves, chopped

2 Tbsp fresh lemon juice

Salt and freshly ground black pepper, to taste

Instructions

1. In a deep pan, place artichokes along with water, oil, cilantro leaves, peppermint, lemon juice, and garlic.

2. Season with salt and pepper to taste and bring to a boil. Reduce heat and simmer artichokes about 15–20 minutes, turning occasionally.

3. Transfer artichokes to a serving platter and drizzle with some of the cooking liquid.

4. Serve.

Servings: 4

Nutrition Facts

Serving size: 1/4 of a recipe (12.8 ounces)

Percent daily values based on the Reference Daily Intake (RDI) for a 2000 calorie diet.

Amount Per Serving

Calories 201.3

Calories From Fat (60%) 121.4

% Daily Value

Total Fat 13.8g 21%

Saturated Fat 1.9g 9%

Cholesterol 0mg 0%

Sodium 149.1mg 6%

Potassium 559.6mg 16%

Total Carbohydrates 11.5g 5%

Fiber 8.3g 33%

Sugar 0.2g

Protein 5.5g 11%

Raw Pistachio Flaxseed Burgers

Ingredients

½ cup ground flaxseed

1 cup pistachio

4 cloves garlic

2 Tbsp lemon juice

2 Tbsp olive oil

sea salt to taste

Instructions

1. Place all ingredients in a food processor; process until well blended.

2. Form two patties with your hands.

3. Serve immediately or refrigerate patties for several hours.

Servings: 3

Cooking Time

Total Time: 15 minutes

Nutrition Facts

Serving size: 1/3 of a recipe (3.7 ounces)

Percent daily values based on the Reference Daily Intake (RDI) for a 2000 calorie diet.

Amount Per Serving

Calories 318.2

Calories From Fat (74%) 235.6

% Daily Value

Total Fat 27.7g 43%

Saturated Fat 3.5g 18%

Cholesterol 0mg 0%

Sodium 1.4mg <1%

Potassium 446.9mg 13%

Total Carbohydrates 13.3g 4%

Fiber 4.3g 17%

Sugar 3.4g

Protein 8.7 g 17%

Olive Crackers with Rosemary

Ingredients

¼ cup chia seeds

½ cup whole flaxseeds

1 large egg

1 egg white

2 sprigs fresh rosemary (cleaned from the steam)

4 Tbsp extra virgin olive oil

sea salt

1 cup of water

Instructions

1. Preheat oven to 300°F.

2. In a bowl, add the flaxseeds and chia, the olive oil and the sea salt to taste.

3. In a separate bowl, first whisk egg, and then add the egg white, the rosemary leaves and the water. Mix well.

4. Add the egg mixture to the flaxseed mixture and mix well until it becomes a homogeneous batter.

5. Let the dough rest for about one hour.

6. On a working surface lay down two pieces of parchment paper.

7. Put the dough on one of the papers and flatten roughly with a spoon.

8. Place the second paper on top and flatten the dough to about 1 inch thick.

9. Finely peel the paper off the top.

10. Cut the dough into squares and place in a baking sheet.

11. Bake for 30 minutes, then peel off the paper and flip over to cool.

Servings: 24

Cooking Time

Inactive Time: 1 hour

Total Time: 45 minutes

Nutrition Facts

Serving size: 1/24 of a recipe (0.7 ounces).

Percent daily values based on the Reference Daily Intake (RDI) for a 2000 calorie diet.

Amount Per Serving

Calories 24.1

Calories From Fat (52%) 12.5

% Daily Value

Total Fat 1.5g 2%

Saturated Fat 0.2g 1%

Cholesterol 7.8mg 3%

Sodium 6.2mg <1%

Potassium 11.9mg <1%

Total Carbohydrates 1.5g <1%

Fiber 1.6g 6%

Sugar 0.0g

Protein 1.1g 2%

Tuna Avocado Burgers

Ingredients

2 cans of tuna

2 Tbsp cream cheese

1 avocado

2 Tbsp grated cheddar cheese

3 Tbsp almond flour

salt, pepper, garlic powder

coconut oil

Instructions

1. Pour the drained tuna into a bowl.

2. Add in the cream cheese, cheddar cheese and spices and mix well. Add sliced avocado to the mixture.

3. Stir the mixture between your hands and make balls. Roll the balls in almond flour.

4. Heat your frying pan at moderate temperature to allow the coconut oil to melt.

5. Cook the tuna burgers three minutes per side (when done, the patties will be browned on the outside).

6. Serve hot.

Servings: 4

Cooking Time

Total Time: 20 minutes

Nutrition Facts

Serving size: 1/4 of a recipe (3.5 ounces)

Percent daily values based on the Reference Daily Intake (RDI) for a 2000 calorie diet.

Amount Per Serving

Calories 194.1

Calories From Fat (61%) 118.4

% Daily Value

Total Fat 13.9g 21%

Saturated Fat 3.1g 15%

Cholesterol 26.2mg 9%

Sodium 201.1mg 8%

Potassium 375.1mg 11%

Total Carbohydrates 5.3g 2%

Fiber 3.7g 15%

Sugar 0.6g

Protein 13.5g 27%

FAT BOMBS (SAVORY AND SWEET)

Cheesy Basil Sausage Fat Bombs

Ingredients

1 Italian sausage, chopped

2 Tbsp yogurt cream cheese, room temperature

2 Tbsp ricotta or cottage cheese

2 Tbsp unsalted butter

1 tsp garlic, minced

1/2 tsp fresh basil (chopped)

4 Tbsp pecan halves, toasted & chopped

parmesan cheese (grated)

Instructions

1. In a bowl, mix chopped sausage, cream cheese, ricotta cheese, butter, chopped basil, garlic and pecans.

2. Make 4 balls, place them on a plate and sprinkle with parmesan cheese.

3. Refrigerate for 4 hours.

4. Serve.

Servings: 4

Cooking Time

Total Time: 10 minutes

Nutrition Facts

Serving size: 1/4 of a recipe (2.1 ounces)

Percent daily values based on the Reference Daily Intake (RDI) for a 2000 calorie diet.

Amount Per Serving

Calories 202.9

Calories From Fat (82%) 167.3

% Daily Value

Total Fat 19.2g 30%

Saturated Fat 7.4g 37%

Cholesterol 47.1mg 16%

Sodium 193.8mg 8%

Potassium 60.9mg 2%

Total Carbohydrates 2.4g <1%

Fiber 0.8g 3%

Sugar 0.5g

Protein 6.6g 13%

Choco-Coco Peppermint Fat Bombs

Ingredients

3 cup melted coconut butter

1 cup finely shredded, unsweetened coconut

3 Tbsp coconut oil, melted

1 tsp pure peppermint extract

2 Tbsp cacao powder

Instructions

1. Mix together melted coconut butter, shredded coconut, 1 tablespoon of coconut oil and peppermint extract.

2. Pour coconut butter mixture into mini muffin tins that have been lined with paper liners. Fill halfway.

3. Place in refrigerator and allow to harden for about 15 minutes.

4. In a bowl, mix together 2 tablespoons coconut oil and cacao powder.

5. Remove muffin tin from refrigerator and top each muffin with chocolate mixture.

6. Return to refrigerator until the chocolate has set.

7. Serve.

Servings: 8

Nutrition Facts

Serving size: 1/8 of a recipe (1.6 ounces)

Percent daily values based on the Reference Daily Intake (RDI) for a 2000 calorie diet.

Amount Per Serving

Calories 124.2

Calories From Fat (97%) 120.2

% Daily Value

Total Fat 13.6g 21%

Saturated Fat 11.0g 55%

Cholesterol 0mg 0%

Sodium 89.6mg 4%

Potassium 33.5mg <1%

Total Carbohydrates 1.3g <1%

Fiber 0.7g 3%

Sugar 0.2g

Protein 0.4g <1%

Coconut Fat Bombs

Ingredients

1/3 cup coconut oil, melted

1 Tbsp shredded coconut

1/3 cup coconut butter, softened

1 tsp granulated sweetener of choice, to taste

Instructions

1. Prepare ice cube trays.

2. Mix all the ingredients in a deep bowl until your natural sweetener is completely dissolved.

3. Pour batter into ice cube trays.

4. Place in refrigerator for two minutes.

5. Serve and enjoy!

Servings: 8

Cooking Time

Total Time: 5 minutes

Nutrition Facts

Serving size: 1/8 of a recipe (1.3 ounces)

Percent daily values based on the Reference Daily Intake (RDI) for a 2000 calorie diet.

Amount Per Serving

Calories 161.2

Calories From Fat (92%) 148.7

% Daily Value

Total Fat 16.9g 26%

Saturated Fat 13.5g 68%

Cholesterol 20.3mg 7%

Sodium 21.2mg <1%

Potassium 5.8mg <1%

Total Carbohydrates 3.0g <1%

Fiber 0.1g <1%

Sugar 0.3g

Protein 0.2g <1%

Macadamia Fat Bombs

Ingredients

3 Tbsp macadamia nuts

5 Tbsp cocoa powder, unsweetened

½ cup coconut oil

2 Tbsp granulated stevia (or sweetener to your choice)

coarse sea salt, to taste

Instructions

1. Melt the coconut oil in a saucepan. Add cocoa powder and the sweetener of your choice.

2. Mix and remove from heat. Add in the chopped nuts and mix well.

3. Pour cocoa and nuts mixture into silicone molds about 3/4 full.

4. Refrigerate for several hours until complctcly hardened.

5. Before serving, remove from silicone molds and place on a serving dish.

6. Serve and enjoy!

Servings: 8

Cooking Time

Total Time: 20 minutes

Nutrition Facts

Serving size: 1/8 of a recipe (1 ounces)

Percent daily values based on the Reference Daily Intake (RDI) for a 2000 calorie diet.

Amount Per Serving

Calories 201.5

Calories From Fat (94%) 188.8

% Daily Value

Total Fat 22.1g 34%

Saturated Fat 13.3g 67%

Cholesterol 0mg 0%

Sodium 1.2mg <1%

Potassium 90.6mg 3%

Total Carbohydrates 3.4g 1%

Fiber 2.0g 8%

Sugar 0.5g

Protein 1.5g 3%

Nutmeg and Cinnamon Fat Bombs

Ingredients

½ cup butter

1/3 cup shredded coconut, unsweetened

1 pinch ground nutmeg

2 pinches ground cinnamon

1 tsp vanilla extract

Instructions

1. Place the butter in a bowl and let melt to room temperature.

2. In a separate bowl, mix together butter, half of the shredded coconut, nutmeg and cinnamon.

3. Make several small-sized balls. Roll in the shredded coconut.

4. Store in refrigerator or freezer for several hours.

Servings: 6

Cooking Time

Total Time: 10 minutes

Nutrition Facts

Serving size: 1/6 of a recipe (0.9 ounces)

Percent daily values based on the Reference Daily Intake (RDI) for a 2000 calorie diet.

Amount Per Serving

Calories 136.6

Calories From Fat (99%) 135.1

% Daily Value

Total Fat 15.4g 24%

Saturated Fat 9.7g 49%

Cholesterol 40.7mg 14%

Sodium 2.1mg <1%

Potassium 5.4mg <1%

Total Carbohydrates 0.1g <1%

Fiber 0.1g <1%

Sugar 0.1g

Protein 0.2g <1%

Rich Bacon Fat Bombs

Ingredients

½ cup butter

4 strips bacon, sliced into small strips

1 ½ green onion, finely diced

2 tsp Worcestershire for steaks

½ tsp black pepper

2 slices bacon, crumbled

Instructions

1. Melt 1 tablespoon butter in a frying pan on medium heat and add in bacon pieces.

2. Add in finely diced onion and fry until onion and bacon are crispy.

3. Set aside and cool to room temp.

4. Add softened butter to a large mixing bowl.

5. Add in bacon and onions, Worcestershire for steaks, and pepper.

6. Use the electric mixer and cream together all ingredients. Roll in the crumbled bacon.

7. Place in refrigerator for 4 hours.

Servings: 6

Cooking Time

Total Time: 15 minutes

Nutrition Facts

Serving size: 1/6 of a recipe (3.2 ounces)

Percent daily values based on the Reference Daily Intake (RDI) for a 2000 calorie diet.

Amount Per Serving

Calories 323.6

Calories From Fat (89%) 289.5

% Daily Value

Total Fat 32.5g 50%

Saturated Fat 15.4g 77%

Cholesterol 66.5mg 22%

Sodium 336.2mg 14%

Potassium 143.9mg 4%

Total Carbohydrates 3.6g 1%

Fiber 0.6g 2%

Sugar 1.5g

Protein 4.9g 10%

Savory Eggs and Lemongrass Fat Bombs

Ingredients

3 cups coconut oil

2 Tbsp organic butter

4 Tbsp cream cheese

3 slices crumbled bacon

4 whole eggs (boiled)

4 egg yolks (boiled)

1 stalk lemongrass

1 tsp freshly grated ginger

1 tsp fresh cilantro, chopped

zest of 1 lime

½ tsp fresh cilantro

1 tsp salt

Instructions

1. Place eggs in a pot and cover with water; for hardboiled eggs, you will need 10-12 minutes.

2. When done, let cool several minutes. Peel the eggs.

3. In a blender, place the coconut oil, organic butter, cream cheese, eggs, yolks, bacon, lemongrass, ginger, lime zest, cilantro and salt. Blend until smooth.

4. Make balls and place in a freezer overnight.

5. Serve.

Servings: 8

Cooking Time

Total Time: 20 minutes

Nutrition Facts

Serving size: 1/8 of a recipe (3.1 ounces)

Percent daily values based on the Reference Daily Intake (RDI) for a 2000 calorie diet.

Amount Per Serving

Calories 342.0

Calories From Fat (91%) 311.6

% Daily Value

Total Fat 35.6g 55%

Saturated Fat 23.9g 120%

Cholesterol 204.4mg 68%

Sodium 315.7mg 13%

Potassium 81.1mg 2%

Total Carbohydrates 0.8g <1%

Fiber 0.0g <1%

Sugar 0.3g

Protein 6.4g 13%

Speedy Pepperoni Fat Bombs

Ingredients

4 slices pepperoni sausages

3 slices pancetta bacon

1/2 cup yogurt cream cheese

1 chili pepper (or jalapeno)

hot paprika (or smoked paprika)

1/2 tsp dried basil

1/4 tsp onion powder

1/4 tsp garlic powder

salt and pepper to taste

Instructions

1. In a bowl, mix all ingredients – chopped pepperoni sausages, pancetta bacon, cream cheese, pepper, spices – and add salt to taste.

2. Mix with the spoon to get a compact mixture.

3. Make 6 balls and refrigerate for 4 hours.

4. Serve.

Servings: 6

Cooking Time

Total Time: 15 minutes

Nutrition Facts

Serving size: 1/6 of a recipe (3.1 ounces)

Percent daily values based on the Reference Daily Intake (RDI) for a 2000 calorie diet.

Amount Per Serving

Calories 150.8

Calories From Fat (77%) 116.2

% Daily Value

Total Fat 13.2g 20%

Saturated Fat 5.5g 28%

Cholesterol 47.8mg 16%

Sodium 361.5mg 15%

Potassium 53.6mg 2%

Total Carbohydrates 2.5g <1%

Fiber 0.4g 2%

Sugar 0.6g

Protein 6.4g 13%

Victory Fat Bombs

Ingredients

½ cup cream cheese

¼ cup ghee

3 Tbsp mayonnaise

4 Tbsp crumbled bacon

1 Tbsp fresh herbs, finely chopped

salt and pepper to taste

grated cheese

Instructions

1. In a food processor mix cream cheese, ghee, mayonnaise and fresh herbs.

2. Place the cheese mass in a bowl and add in the crumbled bacon.

3. Stir lightly with the spoon. Roll in grated cheese.

4. With your hands create 6 balls and refrigerate them for 3 hours.

Servings: 6

Cooking Time

Total Time: 10 minutes

Nutrition Facts

Serving size: 1/6 of a recipe (2.3 ounces)

Percent daily values based on the Reference Daily Intake (RDI) for a 2000 calorie diet.

Amount Per Serving

Calories 210.8

Calories From Fat (87%) 182.7

% Daily Value

Total Fat 20.5g 32%

Saturated Fat 7.9g 39%

Cholesterol 40.4mg 13%

Sodium 325.4mg 14%

Potassium 80.0mg 2%

Total Carbohydrates 2.7g <1%

Fiber 0g 0%

Sugar 1.1g

Protein 4.2g 8%

Wacky Eggs Fat Bombs

Ingredients

6 fresh eggs

4 slices crumbled bacon

2 Tbsp coconut oil

1 Tbsp butter

2 oz cream cheese, softened

1/4 cup shredded Monterey Jack cheese

spices: garlic powder, onion powder, ground pepper, salt, parsley, basil, etc.

coconut flakes, unsweetened

Instructions

1. In small bowl, set aside the butter and oil together to melt at room temperature.

2. Whisk the eggs in a deep bowl. Add spices of your preference.

3. Heat the butter in a non-stick skillet over medium heat. Cook the eggs just for a while, switching off burner before completely done.

4. Put scrambled, slightly cooked eggs into another large bowl. Put in your cheeses and mix. Add bacon and stir.

5. Add the melted butter and coconut oil. Stir thoroughly.

6. Make into balls and roll into coconut flakes.

7. Freeze for about 30 minutes, or refrigerate for 4-5 hours.

Servings: 8

Cooking Time

Total Time: 10 minutes

Nutrition Facts

Serving size: 1/8 of a recipe (2.2 ounces)

Percent daily values based on the Reference Daily Intake (RDI) for a 2000 calorie diet.

Amount Per Serving

Calories 207.2

Calories From Fat (84%) 174.2

% Daily Value

Total Fat 19.6g 30%

Saturated Fat 9.6g 48%

Cholesterol 133.7mg 45%

Sodium 240.6mg 10%

Potassium 91.9mg 3%

Total Carbohydrates 0.6g <1%

Fiber 0g 0%

Sugar 0.4g

Protein 7.1g 14%

KETO SWEETS

Buckwheat Muffins with Nuts

Ingredients

2 ½ cups buckwheat flour

1 ½ cups walnuts, chopped

½ cup sweetener of your choice

4 Tbsp extra virgin olive oil

1 tsp pure vanilla extract

2 tsp baking powder

1 tsp baking soda

Instructions

1. Preheat oven to 345°F.

2. In a small bowl, whisk olive oil, sweetener of your choice and vanilla.

3. In a separate bowl, combine buckwheat flour, baking powder and baking soda. Add in chopped walnuts and toss to coat.

4. Add olive oil mixture to the flour mixture and stir slightly.

5. Spoon the batter into 12 muffin cups, filling 3/4 full.

6. Bake about 20 minutes. Allow to cool and serve.

Servings: 12

Cooking Time

Total Time: 30 minutes

Nutrition Facts

Serving size: 1/12 of a recipe (1.9 ounces)

Percent daily values based on the Reference Daily Intake (RDI) for a 2000 calorie diet.

Amount Per Serving

Calories 270.4

Calories From Fat (52%) 139.8

% Daily Value

Total Fat 16.5g 25%

Saturated Fat 1.6g 8%

Cholesterol 0mg 0%

Sodium 187.1mg 8%

Potassium 204.7mg 6%

Total Carbohydrates 14.2g 6%

Fiber 4.4g 18%

Sugar 1.7g

Protein 7.8g 16%

Keto Flaxseed Pancakes

Ingredients

½ cup ground flax seed meal

2 eggs

2 Tbsp butter, melted

¼ cup heavy cream

3 Tbsp cottage cheese

¼ tsp baking powder

olive oil for frying

Instructions

1. In a deep bowl, mix all ingredients together.

2. Heat the oil in a frying pan. Fry pancakes 2 minutes, flipping when bubbles appear in the middle and the edges turn slightly dry.

3. Cook one minute more on the other side.

4. Serve hot with your favorite cheese and enjoy!

Servings: 6

Nutrition Facts

Serving size: 1/6 of a recipe (1.8 ounces)

Percent daily values based on the Reference Daily Intake (RDI) for a 2000 calorie diet.

Amount Per Serving

Calories 154.8

Calories From Fat (73%) 112.5

% Daily Value

Total Fat 13.0g 20%

Saturated Fat 4.7g 23%

Cholesterol 80.3mg 27%

Sodium 91.5mg 4%

Potassium 143.4mg 4%

Total Carbohydrates 4.5g 2%

Fiber 3.5g 14%

Sugar 0.7g

Protein 6.1g 12%

Mirky Choco Truffles

Ingredients

3 cups almond flour

1 Tbsp flaxseed meal

1 Tbsp cocoa butter

5 Tbsp butter

1 Tbsp coconut oil

1 Tbsp sweetener of your choice

2 tsp vanilla extract

1 cup dark chocolate chips

chopped almonds

pinch of salt

Instructions

1. Combine butter, coconut oil, sweetener, vanilla, almond flour, flaxseed meal and salt in a large bowl.

2. With your hands knead the mixture until all ingredients are incorporated well.

3. Make balls and place them on a sheet of parchment paper; refrigerate for one hour.

4. In a double boiler, melt dark chocolate chips with the cocoa butter.

5. Dip each truffle in the melted chocolate, and place them back on the pan with parchment paper.

6. Refrigerate until the chocolate is completely firm. Serve!

Servings: 14

Cooking Time

Total Time: 50 minutes

Nutrition Facts

Serving size: 1/14 of a recipe (0.9 ounces)

Percent daily values based on the Reference Daily Intake (RDI) for a 2000 calorie diet.

Amount Per Serving

Calories 112.6

Calories From Fat (74%) 82.8

% Daily Value

Total Fat 9.9g 15%

Saturated Fat 2.5g 13%

Cholesterol 0mg 0%

Sodium 19.7mg <1%

Potassium 88.2mg 3%

Total Carbohydrates 5.0g 2%

Fiber 1.3g 5%

Sugar 1.1g

Protein 2.7g 5%

Peanut Butter Ice Cream

Ingredients

½ cup peanut butter, unsweetened

2 ½ cups whipped cream

9 oz cream cheese

1 tsp organic vanilla extract

½ cup sweetener of your choice

peanuts

Instructions

1. Mix all ingredients with an electric mixer until combined well. Adjust sweetener.

2. Pour mixture into a container and freeze for 2 hours.

3. Transfer ice cream mixture into a bowl and beat well with an electric mixer to avoid ice cream crystallization.

4. Freeze again for several hours.

5. Top with peanuts if desired.

6. Serve and enjoy!

Servings: 6

Cooking Time

Preparation Time: 15 minutes

Nutrition Facts

Serving size: 1/6 of a recipe (3.7 ounces)

Percent daily values based on the Reference Daily Intake (RDI) for a 2000 calorie diet.

Amount Per Serving

Calories 389.2

Calories From Fat (69%) 267.4

% Daily Value

Total Fat 31.0g 48%

Saturated Fat 13.9g 70%

Cholesterol 65.8mg 22%

Sodium 267.8mg 11%

Potassium 236.6mg 7%

Total Carbohydrates 21.6g 7%

Fiber 1.3g 5%

Sugar 16.7g

Protein 9.0g 18%

Three Ingredients Mango Cream

Ingredients

2 cups frozen mango

¾ cup heavy cream

10 drops sweetener of your choice

Instructions

1. Add the mango to a high speed blender and beat until it reaches a creamy consistency.

2. Add the heavy cream and continue to whip.

3. Freeze in container for 2 hours.

4. Serve.

Servings: 3

Cooking Time

Preparation Time: 10 minutes

Nutrition Facts

Serving size: 1/3 of a recipe (4.9 ounces)

Percent daily values based on the Reference Daily Intake (RDI) for a 2000 calorie diet.

Amount Per Serving

Calories 169.1

Calories From Fat (60%) 100.7

% Daily Value

Total Fat 11.5g 18%

Saturated Fat 7.0g 35%

Cholesterol 40.9mg 14%

Sodium 12.5mg <1%

Potassium 207.2mg 6%

Total Carbohydrates 12.3g 6%

Fiber 1.8g 7%

Sugar 7.1g

Protein 1.5g 3%

Total Minty Ice Cream

Ingredients

2 cups whipping cream

1 cup almond milk

4 egg yolks

5 drops green food coloring

¼ cup fresh mint leaves, or more to taste

1 tsp mint extract

1 tsp stevia powder (or sweetener of your choice)

Instructions

1. Microwave whipping cream and almond milk in microwave-safe bowl for 2 minutes.

2. In another bowl, combine all other ingredients. Add to heated whipped cream and stir until combined well.

3. Heat the mixture in a saucepan until thickened (but be very careful not to overcook it).

4. Strain into a bowl and chill for 30 minutes. Beat well with an electric mixer. Chill overnight in the fridge.

5. Serve in chilled glasses and enjoy.

Servings: 8

Cooking Time

Preparation Time: 20 minutes

Nutrition Facts

Serving size: 1/8 of a recipe (1.5 ounces)

Percent daily values based on the Reference Daily Intake (RDI) for a 2000 calorie diet.

Amount Per Serving

Calories 138.6

Calories From Fat (88%) 121.8

% Daily Value

Total Fat 13.8g 21%

Saturated Fat 8.0g 40%

Cholesterol 131.3mg 44%

Sodium 16.7mg <1%

Potassium 42.9mg 1%

Total Carbohydrates 2.1g <1%

Fiber 0.2g <1%

Sugar 0.8g

Protein 2.1g 4%